# Rapid Weight Loss Paleo Recipes for Begginers

*by*

**YO MYUNG**

# Simplest Paleo Recipes That Taste Amazing

## Table of Content

Table of Content

Introduction

Quick and Easy Paleo Meal Planning

Paleo Diet Recipes

    Cooking Directions:

    Ingredients:

    Directions:

    Ingredients:

Easy paleo recipes

Quick and Easy Paleo Recipes

    Blueberry Muffin Energy Balls

    Sweet and Spicy Paleo Chicken Fingers

    Avocado Egg Salad Without Mayo

    Cauliflower Fried Rice

# Simplest Paleo Recipes That Taste Amazing

Three Ingredient Paleo Flatbread

The Paleo Dieter Eats Breakfast

   Ingredients:

   Directions:

   Paleo Vaninut Milk Recipe:

   Ingredients:

   Directions:

A Paleo Diet Recipe Anyone Can Make!

   Mayo Free Chicken Salad for a Paleo Diet

   Paleo Chicken Thighs

Paleo Meals You Can Make

Making A Great Paleo Recipe

Delicious Paleo Meatloaf Recipes

   Ingredients:

   Paleo Meat Loaf With Mushrooms

   Ingredients

# Simplest Paleo Recipes That Taste Amazing

Delicious Paleo Late Night Snack Ideas

    Fruit and nut bars

    Vegetables

    Fruit

    Miscellaneous

Paleo Recipe Essentials

    healthfulness

    efficiency

Conclusion

# Simplest Paleo Recipes That Taste Amazing

## Introduction

The Paleo Diet, also called the paleolithic or caveman diet, consists of recipes that are natural such as meat, fish, fruit, vegetables, and nuts. These were the foods that sustained people for years and kept us healthy, physically fit and full of energy; people were strong and thriving. But, something happened that caused our eating habits to change.

Agriculture was introduced to your lifestyle. With the introduction of agriculture, came the introduction of sugar laden, highly processed foods such as wheat flour and high fructose corn syrup. The fast, convenient foods that we are so used to eating, are toxic for our bodies and cause many diseases such as cancer, diabetes, auto immune diseases and more.

# Simplest Paleo Recipes That Taste Amazing

## Quick and Easy Paleo Meal Planning

So you have decided to kick wheat, grains and refined sugar to the curb and adopt a Paleo approach to eating. Or perhaps you have already gone Primal, but are frustrated with what appears to be a total lack of recipes for the food that you can and want to eat. This page will help you learn how to make Paleo meal planning easy and full of the foods you enjoy.

Most of us grew up with the good old food pyramid, which had grains at the bottom. At home, our dinners were laid on a nice mattress of white rice or spaghetti. Otherwise, every meal was divided into three parts; the meat, the veggies, and the starch. The starch usually meant potatoes, rice, or those noodles you made from a packet. It's what we knew, it's what our parents knew, and that was that.

Things have changed a lot. Over the past decade or so, it feels like we have seen a big shift in our approach to food. Now we are starting to rebuild that pyramid, and grains are no longer seen as the perfect base. We are noticing that grains can have a negative effect of some people, and they have no choice but to rebuild their personal food pyramid.

# Simplest Paleo Recipes That Taste Amazing

Some people have chosen to remove the grains entirely in their quest to optimal health, myself included (with certain exceptions - I am not committed enough to be a purist). Many people have achieved positive results by switching to a Paleo diet some or all of the time. The foods that are Paleo change depending on who you ask, but the things most can agree on include:

Fresh fruits and vegetables - most are fine, but a few kinds, such as potatoes, are avoided

Meat and eggs - grass-fed and organic are preferred

Animal and other good fats - choose high-quality animal fats and oils from good sources, such as coconut, avocado, and olive oils

Nuts and seeds (but not peanuts, which are of course, not really nuts)

That is by no means a complete guide to what you can eat, but I am going to have to defer to actual experts on a lot of this. My go-to for Paleo advice is Mark's Daily Apple, which is an excellent resource for those who follow a Paleo or Primal lifestyle.

# Simplest Paleo Recipes That Taste Amazing

So with all that in mind, how do we go about revising our plates when we've taken out 33%-50+% of the stuff we used to pile on it?

Here is a simple guideline for planning Paleo meals.

Take your plate and fill it like this:

1/3 Hearty Vegetables (such as squashes and sweet potatoes - the vegetables that are substantial and add body to a meal)

1/3 Super Vegetables (this is where you load up on nutrient-dense vegetables, such as dark greens or brightly colored tomatoes and peppers)

1/3 Meat (lean protein is good, but a little extra fat is okay here, since it helps keep you feeling full long after the meal)

That is it.

Now it is easy to use this principle to come up with dozens of meals.

# Simplest Paleo Recipes That Taste Amazing

You could set up your Paleo meal plan strategy by making lists of your favorite foods for each category and matching them up.

Starchy Vegetables

Sweet Potato

Acorn Squash

Rutabaga

Carrots

Beets

Super Vegetables

Zucchini

Tomato

Cabbage

Kale

Broccoli

Protein

Eggs

Ground Beef

Pork Chops

# Simplest Paleo Recipes That Taste Amazing

Chicken Legs

Tilapia Filets


Tip: Consider putting ingredients together than pair well or could be cooked together.


For example, you could place cubes of chuck steak in a slow cooker with chunks of butternut squash and pearl onions and celery (there is no limit to how many Super Vegetables you can use). Add some broth, tomato paste, garlic, thyme, salt and pepper, and there you have it!


Avoiding Carbs or Starchy Vegetables?


It should be noted that you don't have to put every category on your plate. For example, if you are trying to avoid vegetables that are high in carbs or sugar (such as sweet potatoes), you could just skip that category and just double up on the Super Vegetables.


Paleo meal planning can be a challenge at times, but if you follow this simple food matching approach and include the healthy foods that you enjoy, it can be.

# Simplest Paleo Recipes That Taste Amazing

## Paleo Diet Recipes

Paleo Diet recipes only include food combinations that are natural, tasty and without toxins including the following:

Egg Drop Soup - Simple yet nutritious Asian inspired soup.

Ingredients:

-2 eggs

-1 egg yolk

-1/4 tsp of salt

-2 tbsp fresh chopped chives

-1/8 tsp of ground ginger

-3 cups of chicken broth

### Cooking Directions:
1. Pour chicken broth into a pot. Medium temp.

2. Add chives, ginger and salt into the pot

3. Mix the eggs

# Simplest Paleo Recipes That Taste Amazing

4. Once broth and spices are boiling, slowly pour the eggs into the pot

Stuffed Pork Tenderloin - Scrumptious piece of pork stuffed with artichoke hearts and sun-dried tomatoes.

## Ingredients:

-1 2lb pork tenderloin

-1 egg

-Sea Salt

Stuffing Ingredients:

-1/2 medium onion, diced

-1/8 fresh thyme, finely chopped

-1/2 fresh sage, finely chopped

-2 large artichoke hearts, diced

-6 sun-dried tomatoes, diced

-2 cloves garlic, finely diced

-A couple tsp of butter or coconut oil

-1/8 tsp nutmeg

# Simplest Paleo Recipes That Taste Amazing

-Sea salt

## Directions:

1. Put all the stuffing ingredients into a pan with medium heat. Saute for about 4 minutes or until the onions are a little golden. Remove it from heat and let it cool down completely.

2. Cut a seam through the center of each piece for the stuffing. Spread butter and salt over it. Place meat in a baking pan.

3. Pre-heat your oven at about 450F.

4. Once the stuffing has cooled down completely, mix in an egg and whisk away.

5. Stuff the meat with your stuffing.

6. Put the stuffed pork into the oven and it will be ready in about 30 minutes.

# Simplest Paleo Recipes That Taste Amazing

Chocolate Cranberry Pie - A Paleo berry-licious treat that you don't have to feel guilty about.

## Ingredients:

Crust Ingredients:

-2 cups of almond flour

-1 egg

-2 tbsp of coconut oil

-1/2 tsp salt

Filling & Topping Ingredients:

-18 oz of frozen cranberries

-1/2 cup of coconut milk

-8 oz of 70% cocoa

Directions:

1. Preheat your oven at 375F.

# Simplest Paleo Recipes That Taste Amazing

2. Put your crust ingredients in a blender. Blend it until you get a crumbly dough texture

3. Lightly grease a pie baking dish and put the dough in it. Firmly press the dough to completely and evenly cover the surface of the entire pan.

4. Put the crust in the oven for about 15 minutes. Let it began to turn golden brown.

5. While the crust is cooking, put the milk in a small pot and bring it to a simmer.

6. Once the it starts to simmer take if off the heat right away and pour the chocolate into the pot. Mix it until completely melted. This is your filling.

7. Once the crust is ready take it out of the oven, pour your filling into the crust.

8. Put the pie in the fridge for at least 2 hours.

# Simplest Paleo Recipes That Taste Amazing

9. Put frozen cranberries in the oven. Bake for about 10 minutes. Once the berries have started to soften take them out the oven and put them in the fridge as well for about 1 hour.

10. Once the crust and filling is nice and solid and the berries are nice and cool, pour them on top of your chocolate filling.

With mouth-watering recipes like this, no one would ever feel like they were missing out. Paleo Diet recipes make it easy for you to incorporate a healthy diet into your life without ever feeling deprived or bored.

Since we have to eat right to take care of our bodies, we may as well enjoy doing it....right

# Simplest Paleo Recipes That Taste Amazing

## Easy paleo recipes

### Guacamole

It's a perfect vehicle for healthy fats and all the other good stuff that you'll find in an avocado. It's delicious scooped over a salad, used as a dip for raw vegetable slices, or simply eaten straight off the spoon.

### Roasted Vegetables

The easiest way of dealing with almost any vegetable is to just toss it on a tray with some Paleo cooking fat and roast it until it's soft and delicious. Roasting more assertive vegetables like broccoli or Brussels sprouts brings out their inner sweetness and makes them much more palatable for kids.

### Chicken soup

Chicken soup is "soul food" after a long day. It's a time-honored home remedy for a sniffle or a flu, and it's an ideal way to use

# Simplest Paleo Recipes That Taste Amazing

up any vegetables loitering in your fridge about to go bad. Plus, it's a perfect vehicle for bone broth.

## Coleslaw

Paleo isn't just about huge hunks of meat all the time: your plate should be at least half-full of vegetables! Per serving, cabbage is one of the cheapest vegetables you can buy, and it's also very easy to prepare. You can fry it, roast it, throw it in a soup…or make coleslaw out of it!

## Chili

A big bowl of chili is just the thing to warm up a cold afternoon. It travels well; it freezes well; it reheats beautifully – is there anything it can't do? You can adjust the spice level up or down, depending on your tastes, and you can throw in just about any kind of meat you can think of!

## Roast Chicken

# Simplest Paleo Recipes That Taste Amazing

It's a classic for a reason – affordable, low-effort, and delicious! Many people are intimidated at the thought of cooking a whole bird instead of just the breasts or drumsticks, but it's really not complicated or difficult. Once you do it for the first time, you'll be amazed that you were ever worried about it.

**Crock-Pot Roasts**

Roasts make it easy to stretch a tight budget (especially if you're feeding a crowd). And slow-cookers make it easy to cram home cooking into even the busiest of schedules. Together, they're a match made in heaven.

# Simplest Paleo Recipes That Taste Amazing

## Quick and Easy Paleo Recipes

### Blueberry Muffin Energy Balls

One of the most difficult things that you might face while starting the Paleo life is giving up on sweets. For those of you who have a natural sweet tooth, this task will seem almost impossible in the beginning. However, the great thing about Paleo is that it takes only about a week to acclimatise your taste buds to the new flavours. If you are still looking for a little sweet something once in a while, these blueberry energy balls will definitely do the trick. All it takes are some nuts, blueberries, dates and seasoning. The recipe is very easy to make as it mostly re uires some blending and the result is a great dessert without the harmful ingredients like refined flour or sugar.

### Sweet and Spicy Paleo Chicken Fingers

Have a Paleo party to throw and cannot figure out the menu? These sweet and spicy chicken fingers are a must try. The best thing about them is that they are not filled with the dangerous trans fats that store made fingers have and neither do they have the usual Standard American Diet gunk. The recipe focuses on providing the best taste with maximum nutritive value and this is perfect if you want to impress the guests without worrying too much about the waistline. Simply combine some almond

# Simplest Paleo Recipes That Taste Amazing

flour with some all natural potato starch and coat the chicken fingers after having seasoned them with Paleo seasonings. Switch to baking with a small drizzle of oil to avoid deep frying them and voila! You have the perfect, healthy appetizer.

## Avocado Egg Salad Without Mayo

While the loss of comfort carbs is a huge adjustment for some of us, the better part of following the Paleo lifestyle is the shift to high quality protein and fats. Some of us will find that this shift is a welcome break from the days of low calorie diets that often leave us craving more food. The Paleo nutrition palate is designed to simultaneously provide more satiety and nutrition and it is keeping this in mind that we now present a classic avocado and egg salad recipe. The highlight of this recipe is the lack of mayo, which many might want to avoid due to the trans fat content. All one needs is some mashed avocado, some light seasoning and boiled eggs. Serve them as part of a snack or even as an appetiser to some party and watch them disappear right under your eyes.

## Cauliflower Fried Rice

When it comes to starches, the other thing that many people miss is rice. Since it has been such an integral part of many cultures, a lot of first time Paleo followers cannot get used to

# Simplest Paleo Recipes That Taste Amazing

the shift away from starchy carbs. Fortunately, there is an easy solution to this issue. Using grated cauliflower as a substitute for white rice is not only a smart decision but also a very easy way to include more veggies in the diet. Cook the grated cauliflower with some low carb green bell peppers and shallots and you have the perfect fried rice with none of the unwanted starch.

## Three Ingredient Paleo Flatbread

One of the most serious changes that you will face while giving up the Standard American Diet is the loss of bread or any wheat item. As many of you might be knowing, wheat if full of gluten that is an anti-nutrient which many cause serious intestinal complications. For all those who are looking for the perfect substitute for bread, this Paleo flatbread recipe is a heaven sent. Use them as part of your sandwiches or even as a side to a Paleo salad. These flatbreads are full of protein and high in fibre and nutrition. Coupled with the fact that they are easy to make, this recipe is bound to make your transition into Paleo much smoother.

# Simplest Paleo Recipes That Taste Amazing

## The Paleo Dieter Eats Breakfast

Breakfast is fairly easy to do Paleo - with plenty of eggs and meats to choose from, making a scramble is quick and easy. One of my favorites I call the Frasier breakfast - tossed salad and scrambled eggs (from the Frasier Show theme song).

Another way is to take leftover veggies and sauté them then add your beaten eggs. Either let them set-up (or stick under the broiler) for frittata or stir them up for a paleo version of Migas.

If you eat bacon or ham (with no nitrates, from organically feed animals), you can fry up the meat and cook eggs in the fat. Very tasty!

And, there's always the power smoothie:

Packed with good fats, proteins, antioxidants and flavor, very satisfying and will keep you going for hours. The possibilities are plentiful; don't limit yourself to the basic egg white protein powder and banana. You can throw into the blender:

# Simplest Paleo Recipes That Taste Amazing

Coconut milk, usually a whole can, some coconut cream if you want extra calories and flavor.

Add any whole fresh or frozen fruit. I like frozen berries either mixed or individuals: strawberries, raspberries, blueberries even cranberries (very tangy). The berries add lots of color to the smoothie and antioxidants.

Add one or two whole raw eggs. Don't worry about raw if you use free range, naturally fed organic eggs. Try some duck or ostrich eggs if you can get them from your local co-op or farmer's market. The eggs add protein and fat.

Or, add a spoonful of your favorite nut butter. It will add a subtle taste of the nut to the finished smoothie. If you want crunchy, add the whole nut instead.

Add a spoon of pure vanilla extract and, there you go!

This is a pretty simple recipe, but it's tasty, ◻uick and powerfully good for you.

# Simplest Paleo Recipes That Taste Amazing

But let's be honest; sometimes you really miss pancakes. So here's a way to stay paleo and have your (pan) cakes too!

The Paleo Diet Quick Pancake Recipe:

## Ingredients:

2 Large eggs

½ Cup Cashew Nut Butter

¼ Teaspoon Cinnamon

½ Cup Apple Sauce (sugarless)

½ Teaspoon Vanilla Extract

Coconut oil

## Directions:

Combine ingredients 1 - 5 in a bowl and stir the mixture until smooth.

# Simplest Paleo Recipes That Taste Amazing

Add a little coconut oil to a frying pan - just enough to lightly cover the bottom. Turn the heat on medium. When the oil starts to pop (or a drop of water dances on the surface), pour the batter and spread it into a pancake shape.

Cook for a minute or two, until the edges start to brown and flip to fry the other side.

Serve with a Paleo-friendly topping of your choice (I prefer Blueberries warmed and mashed into a spread) and enjoy!

Add a Paleo breakfast beverage if you're really hungry.

## Paleo Vaninut Milk Recipe:

## Ingredients:

4 Cups of That Coconut Water

1 Cup Raw Almonds

A pinch of sea salt (if you still use salt)

Seeds from 1Vanilla Bean

# Simplest Paleo Recipes That Taste Amazing

¼ Cup of Agave Nectar or honey equivalent.

## Directions:

Put the coconut water and almonds in a blender and run on high until the mixture looks smooth. Use a nut-milk bag or cheesecloth and strain the mixture, disposing of the pulp.

Return the strained milk mixture to the blender and add the sea salt, vanilla bean seeds, and agave nectar and blend at high speed until smooth.

Want more quick, easy and tasty paleo recipes? Visit The Paleo Dieter blog.

The Paleo Diet may be simple but that doesn't mean you have to eat boring food!

# Simplest Paleo Recipes That Taste Amazing

# A Paleo Diet Recipe Anyone Can Make!

In a large number of Paleo Recipes we see Chicken. And for good reason! Chicken has all the characteristics to be a truly Paleo worthy ingredient. It is tasty, easy to cook in multiple ways, and it can be used in a lot of recipes. For every dish there is a Paleo Chicken Recipe available.

I will show you some of my favorite Paleo Chicken Recipes. I love all of these recipes because they are easy to make, don't require a lot of time and are just delicious. They fit right into my busy life. These Chicken Recipes will definitely keep your taste buds interested and will add some nice taste to your Paleo Diet.

## Mayo Free Chicken Salad for a Paleo Diet

This Chicken Salad is without mayo and therefore it is okay for Paleo. Using lettuce to wrap everything up it is a great, easy to eat dish. Because of the honey and nut butter all the components will actually stick together and stay in your wrap. If

# Simplest Paleo Recipes That Taste Amazing

you'd rather not use nuts, you could always add some sunflower seed butter in the recipe.

1 cup chopped chicken 1/4 green apple, chopped small large handful blueberries small handful chopped raw walnuts 3 chopped celery stalks 1 tbs. dried, juice-sweetened cranberries 2 tsp honey 3 tbs. raw almond butter salt, to taste Romaine lettuce leaves, for serving

The preparation for this dish is very easy. Just mix all the ingredients together in a bowl and wrap it in some lettuce leaves for serving.

## Paleo Chicken Thighs

This is a very simple Chicken Recipe. The dish can be pre-made 12 hours before you want to serve it. This way you can prepare everything when you have the time for it and quickly get it on the table when it's dinner time! This dish is sweet and savory, tangy, and packed with umami. The recipe I will show you here is for 4-5 people. Perfect for a family dinner!

1 bunch scallions, trimmed and cut into thirds

2 garlic cloves, minced

# Simplest Paleo Recipes That Taste Amazing

8 slices of fresh ginger, each approximately the size of a quarter

3 tablespoons rice wine vinegar

3 tablespoons macadamia nut oil or fat of choice

1 tablespoon coconut aminos

1 tablespoon Red Boat fish sauce

2 tablespoons honey (or if you're on the Whole30 or avoiding honey, use ½ small apple, peeled, cored, and diced)

½ teaspoon toasted sesame oil

2 teaspoons kosher salt

Freshly ground pepper to taste

4 pounds chicken thighs


The preparation for this dish is very easy! Put everything EXCEPT for the chicken in a blender or food processor. Blend until everything is smooth. Put the chicken in a food bag or bowl and pour the marinade in. You can leave this in the fridge for up to 12 hours. When you are ready for dinner, simply get the chicken thighs out of the bag, pre-heat your over to 400°F and place them on a rack or baking sheet. Put the chickens with their skin down on it. Now you bake the thighs for 40 minutes. Flip them over at 20 minutes. When the skin is crispy and browned your Paleo Chicken will be ready! (To be sure check if the internal temperature is at 165°F).

# Simplest Paleo Recipes That Taste Amazing

## Paleo Meals You Can Make

There has been a growing demand for Paleo recipes because so many people are switching to a Paleo diet. They are very simple to make and people love them. Paleo meals contain meats that you can choose to bake, poach, stew, or sear. Paleo meals also contain a side dish of vegetables. There are so many variations and you can take basic recipes and create delicious meals with the paleo twist.

Steak and eggs is always a crowd favorite. Now you can make an easy Paleo meal that will make your taste buds happy and keep your diet healthy. You can make this popular dish with just a few ingredients. You will use a large steak, two eggs, two to three tablespoons of tallow or ghee, and paprika. The paprika is optional. Heat two tablespoons of tallow or ghee in a pan over medium heat.

If you like paprika, this is the time to use it. Sprinkle on both sides of the steak. Place your steak in the pan and cook for four minutes on each side. This will give you a medium-rare steak. If you like your steak well done, cook a little longer, as needed. Once you have cooked your steak just the way you like it, remove it from the pan. Now you will crack your eggs and place them into the same pan. Cook your eggs until the whites are no longer transparent. All finished! You can dip your steak into the egg yolk if you want an extra special delight.

# Simplest Paleo Recipes That Taste Amazing

If you are a seafood lover, you are in for a treat. The grilled scallops in red pepper sauce is delicious. They are not only scrumptious, but easy to make as well. Again, just a few ingredients are needed. For this dish, you will need twelve large bay scallops, one-tablespoon coconut oil, and one lemon. For the red pepper sauce, you will need one large roasted red pepper, one clove of garlic, juice from half of a lemon, and two tablespoons of olive oil. You start by squeezing lemon juice over the scallops and letting them sit to marinate.

You can create a smooth sauce by putting all the ingredients for the sauce in a food processor and mixing completely. Pour the sauce in a saucepan and place over medium heat. Once the sauce is simmering, use a grill pan and brush it with the coconut oil. When the grill pan is hot, add the scallops, and cook three to four minutes on each side. Once the scallops are finished, place them on a plate and pour the delicious red pepper sauce over them. Your meal is now complete.

Chicken is always a good choice. You can make a very nutritious and satisfying meal with just three ingredients. Chicken legs and angel hair cabbage is very simple to make. You will need chicken legs, green onion, and angel hair cabbage. That is it. Just three ingredients! You will begin by cooking your chicken legs in a small amount of water, over medium-high heat. Remove them from the pan when they are done.

# Simplest Paleo Recipes That Taste Amazing

You have now created a delicious chicken broth from the water that your chicken legs were cooking in. Add the green onion and angel hair cabbage to your chicken broth. You will want to cook your green onions and angel hair cabbage until they are soft, but not mushy. Cook over medium heat. Once completed, add the chicken back on top and you are ready for a delicious meal.

The Paleo diet is so versatile. The possibilities are endless. Many vegetables and meats work with the Paleo diet. If you are able to figure out which recipe you love the most, you can then top it off with a variety of fresh fruits for dessert

# Simplest Paleo Recipes That Taste Amazing

## Making A Great Paleo Recipe

Many people avoid diets if they can. They do not like being told what they can or cannot eat, even if they do need to eat healthier. Even when they turn to the Paleolithic diet, they are a bit leery about flavor and taste of their meals. Luckily, they quickly discover that a Paleo recipe can be as simple or as sophisticated as they want and remain healthy and tasteful.

During the 1970's, a doctor created a diet based on the way people from the Paleolithic period ate. Since there were no conveniences during that time, like prepared foods, they could only consume what they could gather or hunt. That meant that the people during that time ate a diet rich in fruits, vegetables, meats, nuts, roots, and water.

The key to healthy living with this diet is the ingredients. The ingredients are not only healthy, but they are delicious and versatile. You may eat lean meats such as beef, pork and chicken, as well as wild game. Fish and seafood fall high on the list as well. Other key items in the plan are your vegetables, fruits, nuts, seed, and eggs.

The Paleolithic people were around pre-agricultural period, so they did not have the starchy vegetables and legumes of today. But when eaten in moderation, some of today's modern foods

# Simplest Paleo Recipes That Taste Amazing

can be incorporated into your meal plans. Cereal grains, starchy vegetables, dairy foods, legumes, fruit juice, and even a bit of soda can be added as long as you set boundaries.

There are tons of great recipes around to go with this diet plan or you can create your own easily. In fact, many people already create their own recipes without knowing it. A meal of meat and vegetables can be a basic recipe. You can roast your meat, put it in a pan, or use a crock-pot. Your vegetables can be steamed, roasted, boiled, or raw, the choice is all yours.

You do not have to stick with simplicity if you want to impress guests or create something special for the family. You can create your own soup, stew, curries, sauces, salads, and even omelets. Herbs and spices were used at that time, so adding a touch of basil, garlic, ginger, or creating your own vinaigrette easily fits into the diet plan.

Home cooked meals come to the forefront with Paleolithic diet. Using your natural ingredients, you learn to enjoy cooking again. Unlike you, your grandmother did not enjoy the conveniences of buying mayonnaise or salsa in the store and made it. Now you can learn to cook like that and enjoy eating again, especially when you try new things like venison.

# Simplest Paleo Recipes That Taste Amazing

Eating like a caveman can actually be a compliment to those on the Paleolithic diet, and one they will gladly accept. Consuming only what you can hunt and gather is the core to the plan and eating healthy. But you do not have to give up your favorite comfort foods. Just stick with the key ingredients of the plan to turn any recipe into a Paleo recipe.

## Delicious Paleo Meatloaf Recipes

From standard meatloaf to Paleo meatloaf with just a few small changes!

The humble meatloaf is a long time household favourite. Not only is it a fantastic choice for leftovers, but it is reasonably cheap as well as being so simple to prepare. And with a couple of subtle modifications the recipe can be altered enough to be categorized as a fully approved Paleo Meatloaf! If you have actually never tried it before, have a look at the recipes below and see for yourself just what it is you have actually been missing!

As you probably already know, the Paleo diet plan is about enjoying food that is in its natural form and that can either be hunted or gathered. Keeping this in mind, the humble meatloaf

# Simplest Paleo Recipes That Taste Amazing

does not truly take much altering at all so you can feel comfortable in serving up a fully fledged Paleo meatloaf.

There are a few specs that you need to be aware of but the beauty of a Paleo Meatloaf is in its simplicity. It's another one of those meals that taste just as great (some would say even better!) the second time around so don't be afraid to make heaps that will last a few additional meals! As long as you stay away from the non authorized Paleo items such as grains, artificial sweeteners and especially any processed or synthetic foods, you should be right and you can always add many more different but natural ingredients.

First thing to focus on is the main ingredient... the beef for the Paleo meatloaf! If you are lucky or fortunate enough to be able to get your hands on some home grown beef then great! However, most of us still have to purchase our food from the marketplace or grocery store and what you are trying to find there is Organic Beef which has been preferably grass fed - not grain fed.

Next substitute is the breadcrumbs. Now breadcrumbs are normally an essential part of a ⬜uality meatloaf but uh oh... no grains allowed in a Paleo Meatloaf! You can avoid this detail rather effortlessly by grinding up some oatmeal till it looks and feels the same consistency and texture of breadcrumbs.

# Simplest Paleo Recipes That Taste Amazing

Lots of meatloaf recipes call for using tomato sauce, ketchup or catsup. These are also not allowed as they often contain a lot of preservatives, add-ons and also high fructose corn syrup. Some folks following the Paleo meal plan, specifically time poor people, can be easily lured to use these but it is so simple to stay true and make Paleo diet plan friendly catsup... and it's so easy!

All you have to do for your Paleo diet plan friendly catsup is to mix together a 6 ounce can of natural tomato paste with 2 Tbsp of vinegar, 1/4 cup water, 1/2 tsp each of sea salt, ground cloves, and allspice. You're ready to go!

Now... to the recipes!

I have two recipes here for you to choose from. Just choose the one that appears the most appealing to you and get started on a yummy Paleo Meatloaf for you and your family tonight!

Paleo Meatloaf Recipe 1:

# Simplest Paleo Recipes That Taste Amazing

## Ingredients:

2 lbs. lean ground beef

2 eggs

1 tsp of sea salt

1 stalk celery

1 medium sized bell pepper, chopped

1 medium sized onion, sliced

1 teaspoon black pepper

2/3 cup ground oatmeal

1 tsp of thyme

1 teaspoon of garlic

1/2 cup catsup (recipe above)

Toss everything into a large mixing bowl but only use half the catsup as you will require the other half a little later. Mix together thoroughly. When blended, place the mixture into a softly greased pan. Now grab the remaining catsup and spread

# Simplest Paleo Recipes That Taste Amazing

it evenly over the top of the meatloaf. Pop it straight into a 350 degree oven and let it cook for around half an hour.

## Paleo Meat Loaf With Mushrooms

Mushroom fans will enjoy this one! The mushrooms not only contribute to the remarkable taste of this dish but also assist it bind together and all in all, it results in a very filling meal. Either served on its own or with a light side salad it will certainly become a family favourite! This recipe serves 5 Neanderthals!

## Ingredients

2 lb ground beef

1 1/2 tsp sea salt

1 tsp ground black pepper

1 egg

1 medium onion, finely chopped

2 cups white button mushrooms, carefully chopped

1 tsp chili pepper flakes

3 tsp fresh thyme, minced

# Simplest Paleo Recipes That Taste Amazing

1 tsp fresh oregano, minced

3 cloves garlic, minced

1/2 cup homemade ketchup

1 tbsp Paleo cooking fat

Like the first Paleo meatloaf recipe, all the ingredients are blended together, a loaf is formed and then the meatloaf is topped with catsup or homemade tomato sauce then popped in a 350 degree oven for about an hour or until the meat is cooked and not pink in the middle. The only difference in this one is that the mushrooms have to be cooked first. Over a medium heat in a skillet or fry pan, thaw the Paleo cooking fat and simply sauté the mushrooms until soft. This should not take more than 2 or 3 minutes.

So there you have it my friends, 2 different recipes for you to try. There are far more choices of Paleo dinners than people think and I hope that a yummy Paleo meatloaf becomes part of your weekly menu!

# Simplest Paleo Recipes That Taste Amazing

## Delicious Paleo Late Night Snack Ideas

Those who follow the Paleo diet, might end up in a dead end when it comes to snacks recipes. Restrict ingredients might size down the ideas for snacks, especially the Paleo late night snacks.

Everyone has experienced the need for a snack late at night while watching TV or on the computer. The question is: What shall I eat? Although it might sound difficult to figure out, it is rather easy to get a Paleo snack if we have some simple ingredients at home.

### Fruit and nut bars

One of the easiest ways to get a good Paleo late night snack is through fruit and nut bars. They are available in supermarket shelves and ready to be eaten on the spot. Special Paleo packages will provide the necessary nutrients without the need to worry about cooking or getting the Paleo ingredients. Of course fruit and nut bars can also be prepared at home. Almonds, pecans, pistachios, macadamia nuts and honey are some of the necessary ingredients to be used in the preparation. Having pre-made snacks available, is the best way to take care of the stomach late at night.

# Simplest Paleo Recipes That Taste Amazing

## Vegetables

Fully Paleo, vegetables can be eaten in large quantities and they are one of the preferred food in the Paleo diet. Whether it is a carrot, lettuce or tomato, they can be eaten without being cooked; therefore they are an excellent alternative to a Paleo late night snack that may require cooking, or intricate preparation.

## Fruit

Although fruit should be eaten moderately while on a Paleo diet, a little snack does not do any harm. A small banana, kiwi, grapes, pears, apples or strawberries can be eaten without any extra ingredient. However, almond butter or honey can be added for additional flavor.

## Miscellaneous

There are other snacks that can be made by mixing several ingredients like:

Fruit and nut salad: where the taste of fruit is intensified by the

# Simplest Paleo Recipes That Taste Amazing

flavor of several types of nuts. Honey can always be added as a natural sweetener.

Meat and fruit:stuffed dates where almonds, nut butter and bacon are all combined with dates turning this combination into a mixture of flavors and healthy nutrients. Although this recipe has a cooking time of 20 to 25, it is worth every waiting minute. The stuffed dates can be cooked during dinner time and saved for later, already thinking about the late snack that will be needed.

Vegetable Mini Quiche:Eggs, meat and vegetables are the three main ingredients for the mini quiches. Very easy to prepare and with a maximum cooking time of 30 minutes, these mini quiches are terrific snacks that taste even better when they are cold. They can be cooked during lunch or dinner or even overnight. Having them available in the kitchen means being tasty Paleo late night snack ready.

There is an endless list of Paleo late night snacks available. Sometimes we just have to let our imagination wonder and combine different foods to get tasty, healthy and fully Paleo snack recipes. Like in other Paleo recipes, adding a new ingredients or replacing one with a different ingredient is the best option to get a big variety of recipes.

# Simplest Paleo Recipes That Taste Amazing

## Paleo RecipeEssentials

Paleo recipes are easy and have limited ingredients. Recipes are: grain-free, bean-free, potato-free, dairy-free, and sugar-free. Recipes that members of this community take pleasure in are obtainable for you to explore. You'll in addition to take pleasure in making a little of the preferred paleo diet recipes.

### Healthfulness

Healthy, delicious, and simple, the Paleo Diet is the diet we were planned to consume. They include everything from light summer salads to hearty winter soups, all without using any of the unhealthy ingredients that generally lead our favorite dishes. The Paleo Cookbooks clearly show that eating healthy does not in any way have to be boring or tasteless. You will be able to create recipes that help you to stay away from unhealthy sweets and fried foods. A Paleo diet, additionally established as paleolithic diet or caveman diet, is all about natural foods to help achieve excellent healthfulness and a good physi☐ue.

In The Paleo Diet, you'll detect how to improve your health and lose weight by simulating a Paleolithic diet from healthful foods applicable at your local grocery store. Numerous humans experience health benefits within the first week to 10 days after

# Simplest Paleo Recipes That Taste Amazing

using this remarkable diet. every assumption that your vegetarian friends use to avoid meat for health reasons is debunked here. In order to actually lose weight using any diet you need food you like to consume that are nutritious. If you want flavor and healthy all in one shot, the Paleo Recipes are the way to go.

## Efficiency

Uncover how a diet based on lean meats, seafood, fresh fruits, and fresh vegetables can lead to ideal body weight, optimum health, and perfect athletic efficiency. By consuming the foods that we are genetically accustomed to eat, followers of the Paleo Diet are naturally lean, have acne-free skin, improved athletic performance, and are experiencing relief from diversified metabolic-related and autoimmune diseases.

The Paleo Diet for Athletes demonstrates how four principal dietary changes that you will make are ergogenic (performance enhancing) for endurance athletes or for anyone ordinarily wanting to attain in shape. They'll acknowledge the significance of dietary fats whether the consideration is performance, health, longevity, or making your fanny look excellent in a bikini. human beings have followed the paleo diet to lose weight, increase their power, enhance their exercise effectiveness and/or to mainly focus on achieving the very preferred ade☐uately being attainable. It had been proven impressive in bestowing the following benefits specific as increased energy, smoother and fairer skin, stronger immune process and

# Simplest Paleo Recipes That Taste Amazing

exceeding effectiveness. I encourage anyone who wants to lose weight, have more energy, enhance fertility, fuel sports performance or readily be nutritious while having no doubt what foods should be eaten to be healthy to get those recipes now. people have followed the paleo diet to lose weight, increase their power, enhance their exercise efficiency and/or to customarily focus on achieving the very preferred absolutely being attained.

# **Conclusion**

Thank you again for downloading this book!

Finally, if you enjoyed this book, then I'd like to ask you for a favor, would you be kind enough to leave a review for this book on Amazon? It'd be greatly appreciated!

Printed in Great Britain
by Amazon